The Mediterranean DIET Cookbook For Beginners

Change Your Daily Lifestyle with Healthy Delicious and Affordable Mediterranean Recipes.

Angela D. Lovato

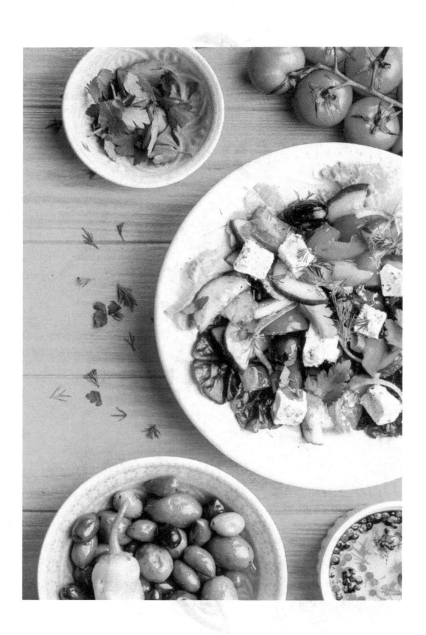

Table of content

MEDITERRANEAN BREAKFAST RECIPE

Mediterranean Frittata

Total time: 25 minutes

Prep time: 10 minutes

Cook time: 15 minutes

Yield: 4 servings

Ingredients

- 3 tbsp. extra virgin olive oil, divided
- 1 cup chopped onion
- 2 cloves garlic, minced
- 8 eggs, beaten
- ¼ cup half-and-half, milk or light cream
- ½ cup sliced Kalamata olives
- ½ cup roasted red sweet peppers, chopped
- ½ cup crumbled feta cheese
- ⅛ tsp. black pepper
- ¼ cup fresh basil
- 2 tbsp. Parmesan cheese, finely shredded
- ½ cup coarsely crushed onion-and-garlic croutons
- Fresh basil leaves, to garnish

Directions

- Preheat your broiler.
- Heat 2 tablespoons of extra virgin olive oil in a broiler-proof skillet set over medium heat; sauté onion and garlic for a few minutes or until tender.
- In the meantime, beat eggs and half-and-half in a bowl until well combined.

- Stir in olives, roasted sweet pepper, feta cheese, black pepper and basil.
- Pour the egg mixture over the sautéed onion mixture and cook until almost set.
- With a spatula, lift the egg mixture to allow the uncooked part to flow underneath.
- Continue cooking for 2 minutes more or until the set.
- Combine the remaining extra virgin olive oil, Parmesan cheese, and crushed croutons in a bowl; sprinkle the mixture over the frittata and broil for about 5 minutes or until the crumbs are golden and the top is set.
- To serve, cut the frittata into wedges and garnish with fresh basil.

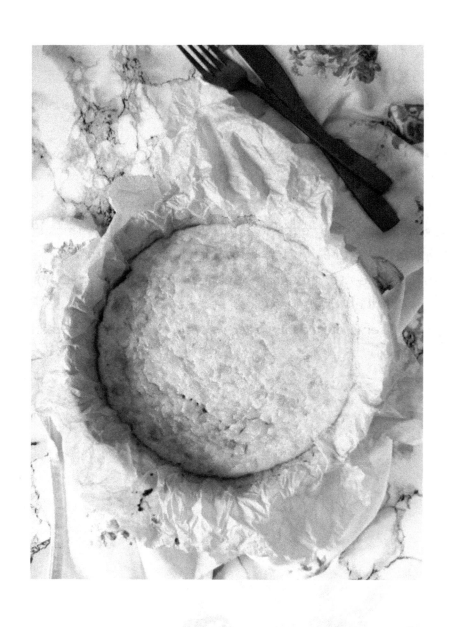

Nutty Banana Oatmeal

Total time: 15 minutes

Prep time: 10 minutes

Cook time: 5 minutes

Yield: 4 servings

Ingredients

- ¼ cup quick cooking oats
- 3 tbsp. raw honey
- ½ cup skim milk
- 2 tbsp. chopped walnuts
- 1 tsp. flax seeds
- 1 banana, peeled

Directions

- In a microwave-safe bowl, combine oats, honey, milk, walnuts, and flaxseeds; microwave on high for about 2 minutes.
- In a small bowl, mash the banana with a fork to a fine consistency; stir into the oatmeal and serve hot.

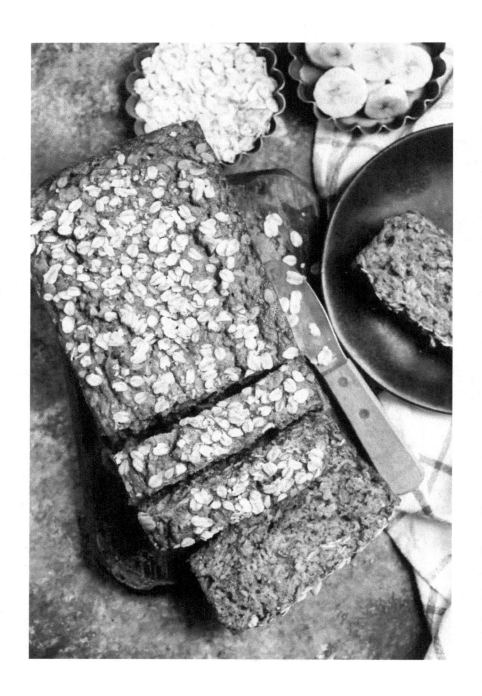

Mediterranean Veggie Omelet

Total time: 40 minutes

Prep time: 15 minutes

Cook time: 25 minutes

Yield: 4 servings

Ingredients

- 1 tbsp. extra virgin olive oil
- 2 cups thinly sliced fresh fennel bulb
- ¼ cup chopped artichoke hearts, soaked in water, drained
- ¼ cup pitted green olives, brine-cured, chopped
- 1 diced Roma tomato
- 6 eggs
- ¼ tsp. sea salt
- ½ tsp. freshly ground black pepper
- ½ cup goat cheese, crumbled
- 2 tbsp. freshly chopped fresh parsley, dill, or basil

Directions

- Preheat your oven to 325°F.
- Heat extra virgin olive oil in an ovenproof skillet over medium heat.
- Sauté fennel for about 5 minutes or until tender.
- Add artichoke hearts, olives, and tomatoes and cook for 3minutes ore or until softened.
- In a bowl, beat the eggs; season with sea salt and pepper.
- Add the egg mixture over the vegetables and stir for about 2 minutes.

- Sprinkle cheese over the omelet and bake in the oven for about 5 minutes or until set and cooked through.
- Top with parsley, dill, or basil.
- Transfer the omelet onto a cutting board, carefully cut into four wedges, and serve immediately.

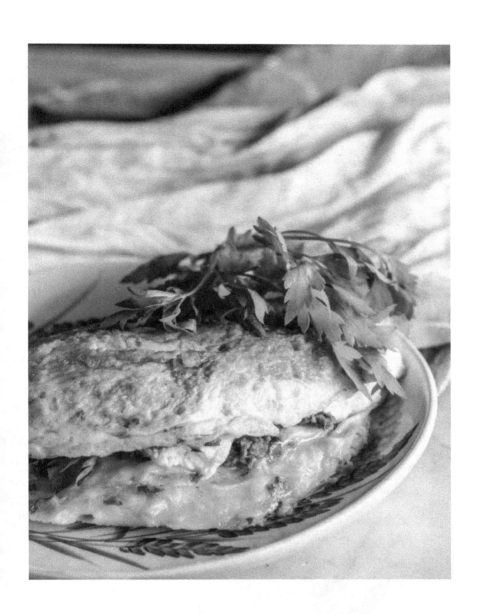

Lemon Scones

Total time: 30 minutes

Prep time: 15 minutes

Cook time: 15 minutes

Yield: 12 servings

Ingredients

- 2 cups plus ¼ cup flour
- ½ tsp. baking soda
- 2 tbsp. sugar
- ½ tsp. sea salt
- ¾ cup reduced-fat buttermilk
- Zest of 1 lemon
- 1 to 2 tsp. freshly squeezed lemon juice
- 1 cup powdered sugar

Directions

- Preheat your oven to 400°F.
- In a food processor, combine 2 cups of flour, baking soda, sugar and salt until well blended.
- Add buttermilk and lemon zest and continue mixing to combine well.
- Sprinkle the remaining flour onto a clean surface and turn out the dough; gently knead the dough at least six times and shape it into a ball.
- Using a rolling pin, flatten the dough into half-inch thick circle.

- Cut the dough into four equal wedges and the cut each into three smaller wedges.
- Arrange the scones on a baking sheet and bake in preheated oven for about 15 minutes or until golden brown.
- Mix together lemon juice and the powdered sugar in a small bowl to make a thin frosting.
- Remove the scones from the oven and drizzle with lemon frosting while still hot.
- Serve right away.

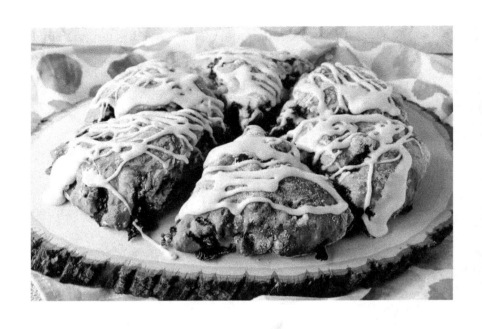

Breakfast Wrap

Total time: 10 minutes

Prep time: 5 minutes

Cooking time: 5 minutes

Yield: 2 servings

Ingredients

- ½ cup fresh-picked spinach
- 4 egg whites
- 2 Bella sun-dried tomatoes
- 2 mixed-grain flax wraps
- ½ cup feta cheese crumbles

Directions

- Cook spinach, egg whites and tomatoes in a frying pan for about 4 minutes or until lightly browned.
- Flip it over and cook the other side for 4 minutes or until almost done.
- Microwave the wraps for about 15 seconds; remove from the microwave, fill each wrap with the egg mixture, sprinkle with feta cheese crumbles and roll up.
- Cut each wrap into two parts and serve.

MEDITERRANEAN LUNCH RECIPE

Maple Pumpkin Pie Buckwheat Groats

Ingredients

- ½ cup raw buckwheat groats
- 2/3 cup unsweetened almond milk beverage
- ½ teaspoon pumpkin pie spice
- 1/8 teaspoon salt
- ½ teaspoon vanilla extract
- 4 teaspoons 100% pure maple syrup

Preparation

- Place groats in a bowl and cover them with water. Place groats in the refrigerator to soak overnight. The next day, drain the groats. It is normal for buckwheat to be somewhat mucilaginous, so groats will be slippery. Rinse well and drain again.
- To a 2-quart saucepan, add the groats, almond milk, pumpkin pie spice, and salt, and whisk to dissolve the spices. Cover and bring to a boil, then reduce heat to a low simmer and cook for 4 minutes. Remove cover and turn heat up to maintain a simmer and cook for an additional 2 minutes, stirring occasionally.
- Remove from the heat and stir in vanilla and maple syrup.

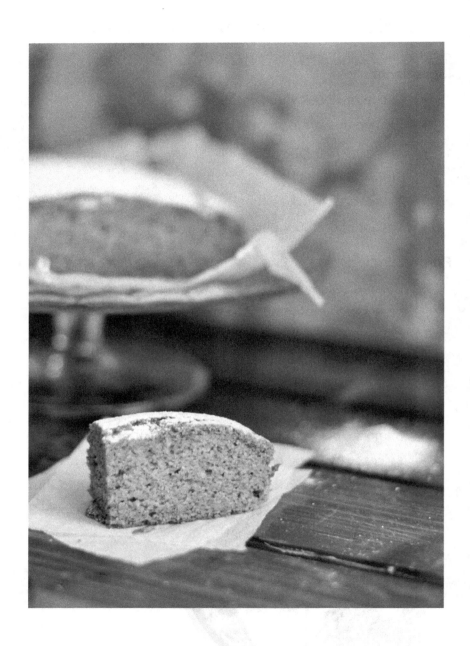

Chicken, Broccoli, and Rice Casserole
Recipe

Ingredients

- 12 ounces boneless, skinless chicken breast
- 1/4 teaspoon sea salt
- 3/4 teaspoon freshly cracked black pepper, divided
- 2 tablespoons olive oil, divided
- 1/2 medium yellow onion, diced
- 2 cloves garlic, minced
- 3 cups frozen broccoli florets
- 1 tablespoon whole wheat flour or all-purpose flour
- 1 1/2 cups skim milk
- 3/4 cups sharp cheddar cheese, freshly grated, divided
- 2 cups cooked whole grain wild rice blend
- Cooking spray
- 1/4 cup whole wheat panko breadcrumbs

Preparation

- Heat oven to 350F. Cut chicken into 1/2-inch cubes. Season with salt and 1/4 teaspoon pepper.
- In a large skillet, heat 1/2 tablespoon of the oil over medium heat. Add chicken and cook, stirring, until chicken is cooked through. Remove chicken to a large bowl.
- In the same skillet, heat another 1/2 tablespoon of oil. Add garlic, onion, and broccoli. Cook, stirring until onion is soft and broccoli is bright green. Pour into bowl with chicken.

- Turn heat to low and add the remaining tablespoon of oil to the skillet. Sprinkle flour over oil and whisk to make a paste. Slowly add milk, whisking to combine. Stir in cheese and remaining 1/2 teaspoon of black pepper. Remove from heat.
- Add rice to chicken and broccoli in the large bowl. Stir to combine. Gently stir in cheese sauce.
- Spray a 9x9-inch baking dish with cooking spray. Spread rice mixture into baking dish. Sprinkle with remaining 1/4 cup of cheese and breadcrumbs.
- Bake 15 to 20 minutes, or until cheese is melted and casserole is bubbly. Remove from the oven and serve hot

Baked Coconut Rice

Ingredients

- 1 tablespoon coconut oil
- 2 cups uncooked brown jasmine rice
- 1 teaspoon salt
- 13.5-ounce can coconut milk
- 2 cups water
- ½ cup slivered fresh pineapple
- ¼ cup toasted coconut flakes
- ¼ cup toasted sliced almonds

Preparation

- Preheat the oven to 375F.
- In a 4-quart ovenproof pot, melt the coconut oil over medium heat on the stovetop. Rinse and drain the rice in a mesh strainer and add it to the coconut oil. Brown the rice, stirring occasionally, for 5 minutes. Add the salt, coconut milk, and water. Bring the rice to a boil.
- Cover the pot tightly with a heavy lid or aluminum foil and place it in the oven. Bake for 35 minutes. Test it to make sure it is almost tender. If it isn't almost tender, add another quarter cup of water and return it to the oven for another 10 minutes. Allow the rice to rest, covered, for 5 more minutes to complete the cooking process. Fluff and serve the rice, garnished with slivered pineapple, coconut flakes, and sliced almonds.

Healthy Butternut Squash Grain Bowl

Ingredients

- 1 cup butternut squash cubes
- 1 teaspoon olive oil
- 1 teaspoon maple syrup
- 1/4 teaspoon cinnamon
- 1/4 teaspoon freshly cracked pepper
- Pinch salt
- 1/4 cup pecans
- 1 cup cooked wild rice
- 2 cups baby spinach or spring mix
- 1 small Honeycrisp apple
- 1/4 cup dried cranberries

Preparation

- Heat oven to 400F. Line a baking sheet with parchment or a silicone baking mat.
- Toss butternut squash with oil, syrup, cinnamon, pepper, and salt. Spread evenly on the baking sheet and roast for 25 to 30 minutes, stirring occasionally.
- Place pecans on a piece of foil or small baking sheet and toast at 400F for 5 to 10 minutes or until fragrant, watching carefully.
- Assemble bowls. Divide rice between two bowls. Add greens, squash, apples, cranberries and toasted pecans.

Low Sodium Garlic Parmesan Popcorn

Ingredients

- 2 teaspoons olive or avocado oil
- 1/4 cup popcorn kernels
- 2 cloves garlic, minced
- 2 tablespoons good quality parmesan cheese, freshly grated
- 1/4 teaspoon garlic powder

Preparation

- Heat oil in the bottom of a small saucepan over medium high heat. Add 2 or 3 kernels to the pan while heating.
- Once kernels start to pop, add remaining popcorn kernels and garlic. Cover the pan and cook, shaking the pan to keep kernels from burning.
- Once kernels have stopped popping, remove from heat and sprinkle the parmesan and garlic powder on top. Shake to coat popcorn evenly, then pour into bowls and enjoy.

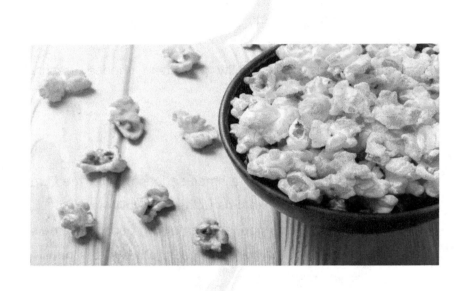

Gluten-Free Coconut Granola

Ingredients

- 3 cups certified gluten-free rolled oats
- ½ cup sweetened shredded coconut
- ¼ teaspoon kosher salt
- 1/3 cup maple syrup
- 1 tablespoon canola oil
- ½ cup sliced almonds
- 1 cup dried cranberries

Preparation

- Preheat oven to 325°F.
- Line a large sheet pan with parchment paper; set aside.
- Combine gluten free oats, coconut, salt, maple syrup, and canola oil in a large bowl.
- Toss ingredients well and pour out onto a prepared baking sheet.
- Bake, stirring occasionally, until golden brown (15 to 20 minutes).
- Remove from oven to cool.
- Once cool, mix in almonds and dried cranberries.
- Enjoy right away or store in an airtight container for up to 2 weeks.

Simple Black Bean and Barley Vegetarian Burritos

Ingredients

- 1/2 cup barley, dry
- 1 tablespoon olive oil
- 1 small onion, chopped
- 1 teaspoon dry garlic
- pinch red pepper flakes
- 1/4 teaspoon cumin
- 1/4 teaspoon salt
- 3 tablespoons tomato paste
- 1 medium carrot, shredded
- 1 15-ounce can black beans
- 6 large whole wheat tortillas (9 or 10 inches across)
- avocado, salsa, shredded cheddar, or sour cream, for garnish and dipping, optional

Preparation

- Prepare barley according to package instructions.
- While barley is cooking, heat up olive oil in a medium-sized pan over medium heat. Add onion, garlic, pepper flakes, cumin, salt, tomato paste, carrot, and black beans. Stir together and let heat for about 5 minutes. Remove from heat and mash the mixture slightly with a fork.
- Once barley is ready, place each tortilla on a separate plate. Divide the barley and black bean mixture into six parts and arrange them towards the middle of each tortilla.

30

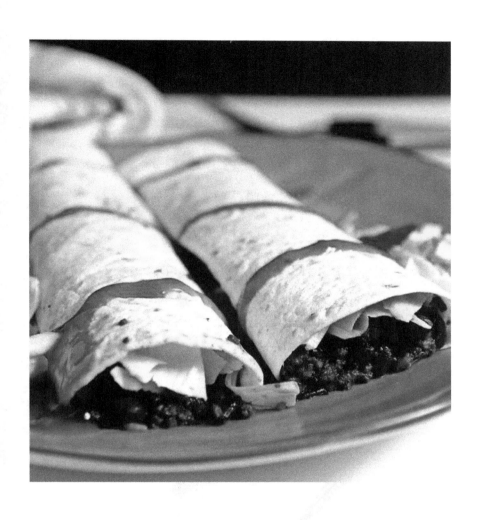

MEDITERRANEAN SALAD RECIPES

Healthy Greek Salad

Total time: 15 minutes

Prep time: 15 minutes

Cook time: 0 minutes

Yield: 6 servings

Ingredients

- 1 small red onion, chopped
- 2 cucumbers, peeled and chopped
- 3 large ripe tomatoes, chopped
- 4 tsp. freshly squeezed lemon juice
- ¼ cup extra virgin olive oil
- 1 ½ tsp. dried oregano
- Sea salt
- Ground black pepper
- 6 pitted and sliced black Greek olives
- 1 cup crumbled feta cheese

Directions

- Combine onion, cucumber, and tomatoes in a shallow salad bowl; sprinkle with lemon juice, extra virgin olive, oregano, sea salt and black pepper.
- Sprinkle the olives and feta over the salad and serve immediately.

Almond, Mint and Kashi Salad

Total time: 1 hour 35 minutes

Prep time: 15 minutes

Cook time: 1 hour

Cooling time: 20 minutes

Yield: 4 servings

Ingredients

- 4 tbsp. extra virgin olive oil, divided, plus more for drizzling
- 1 small onion, finely chopped
- Sea salt, to taste
- Freshly ground black pepper, to taste
- 2 cups water
- 1 cup Kashi 7-Whole Grain Pilaf
- 2 bay leaves
- 3 tbsp. fresh lemon juice
- 5 tbsp. sliced natural almonds, divided
- 8 cherry tomatoes, quartered
- ¼ cup chopped parsley
- ¼ cup chopped fresh mint
- 4 large romaine leaves

Directions

- Heat 2 tablespoons of extra virgin olive oil in a large saucepan set over medium heat.
- Add onion, sea salt and pepper and cook, stirring occasionally, for about 5 minutes or until lightly browned and tender.

- Stir in 2 cups of water, Kashi, bay leaves, sea salt and pepper; bring the mixture to a rolling boil, lower heat to a simmer and cook, covered, for about 40 minutes or until Kashi is tender.
- Transfer to a large bowl and discard bay leaves, and then stir in the remaining extra virgin olive oil, and lemon juice.
- Let sit for at least 20 minutes or until cooled to room temperature.
- Adjust the seasoning if desired and add 4 tablespoons almonds, tomatoes, parsley, and mint; toss to mix well.
- Place one romaine leaf on each of the four plates and spoon the mixture into the center of the leaves; drizzle with extra virgin olive oil and sprinkle with the remaining almonds.

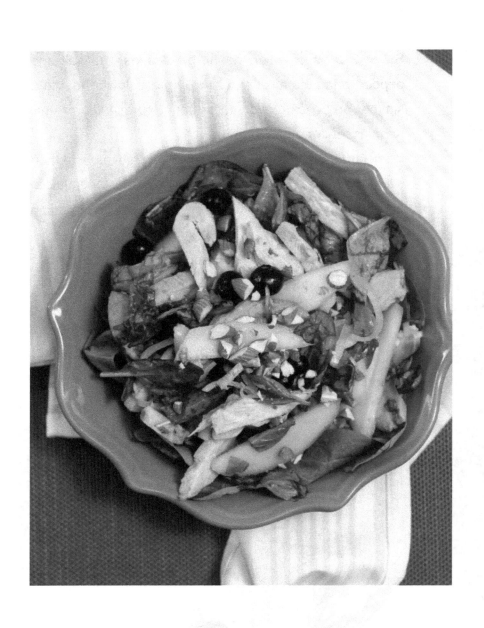

Chickpea Salad

Total time: 1 hour, 20 minutes

Prep time: 10 minutes

Cook time: 40 minutes

Standing time: 30 minutes

Yield: 6 servings

Ingredients

- 1 ½ cups dried chickpeas, soaked and liquid reserved
- 1 ¼ tsp. sea salt, divided
- 1 garlic clove, minced
- 2 tbsp. extra virgin olive oil
- 3 tbsp. sherry vinegar
- 16 crushed whole black peppercorns
- ¾ tsp. dried oregano
- 3 scallions, sliced into ½-inch pieces
- 2 carrots (4 ounces), cut into ½-inch dice
- 1 cup diced green bell pepper
- ½ English cucumber, peeled and diced
- 2 cups halved cherry tomatoes
- 2 tbsp. shredded fresh basil
- 3 tbsp. chopped fresh parsley

Directions

- Combine the chickpeas and soaking liquid in a large pot and season with ¾ teaspoons of sea salt.
- Bring the mixture to a gentle boil over medium heat. Lower heat to a simmer and cook, stirring occasionally, for about

40 minutes or until the chickpeas are tender; drain and transfer to a large bowl.

- In the meantime, mash together garlic and salt to form a paste; transfer to a separate bowl and stir in extra virgin olive oil, vinegar, peppercorns, and oregano to make the dressing.
- Pour the garlic dressing over the chickpeas and let stand for at least 30 minutes, stirring once.
- Toss in scallions, carrots, bell pepper, cucumber, tomatoes, basil, and parsley.
- Serve.

MEDITERRANEAN POULTRY RECIPES

Braised Chicken with Olives

Total time: 1 hour 50 minutes

Prep time: 20 minutes

Cook time: 1 hour 30 minutes

Yield: 4 servings

Ingredients

- 1 tbsp. extra virgin olive oil
- 4 whole skinned chicken legs, cut into drumsticks and thighs
- 1 cup low-sodium canned chicken broth
- 1 cup dry white wine
- 4 sprigs thyme
- 2 tbsp. chopped fresh ginger
- 2 garlic cloves, minced
- 3 carrots, diced
- 1 medium yellow onion, diced
- 3/4¾ cup chickpeas, drained, rinsed
- ½ cup green olives, pitted and roughly chopped
- ⅓ cup raisins
- 1 cup water

Directions

- Preheat your oven to 350°F.
- Heat extra virgin olive oil in a Dutch oven or a large ovenproof skillet over medium heat.

- Add the chicken pieces into the skillet and sauté for about 5minutes per side or until browned and crisped on both sides.
- Transfer the cooked chicken to a plate and set aside.
- Lower heat to medium low and add garlic, onion, carrots, and ginger to the same skillet; cook, stirring, for about 5 minutes or until onion is translucent and tender.
- Stir in water, chicken broth, and wine; bring the mixture to a gentle boil.
- Return the chicken to the pot and stir in thyme.
- Bring the mixture back the boil and cover.
- Transfer to the oven and braise for about 45 minutes.
- Remove the pot from the oven and stir in chickpeas, olives, and raisins.
- Return to oven and braise, uncovered, for 20 minutes more.
- Remove the skillet from oven and discard thyme.
- Serve immediately.

Braised Chicken with Mushrooms and Olives

Total time: 45 minutes

Prep time: 10 minutes

Cook time: 35 minutes

Yield: 4 servings

Ingredients

- 2 ½ pounds chicken, cut into pieces
- Sea salt
- Freshly ground pepper
- 1 tbsp. plus 1 tsp. extra virgin olive oil
- 16 cloves garlic, peeled
- 10 ounces cremini mushrooms, rinsed, trimmed, and halved
- ½ cup white wine
- ⅓ cup chicken stock
- ½ cup green olives, pitted

Directions

- Heat a large skillet over medium-high heat.
- In the meantime, season the chicken with sea salt and pepper.
- Add 1 tablespoon of extra virgin olive oil to the heated skillet and add the chicken, skin side down; cook for about 6 minutes or until browned.
- Transfer to a platter and set aside.

- Add the 1 teaspoon of remaining extra virgin olive oil to the pan and sauté garlic and mushrooms for about 6 minutes or until browned.
- Add wine and bring to a gentle boil, reduce heat and cook for about 1 minute.
- Add the chicken back to the pan and stir in chicken broth and olives.
- Bring the mixture back to a gentle boil, reduce heat and simmer, covered, for about 20 minutes or until the chicken is cooked through.

Chicken with Olives, Mustard Greens, and Lemon

Total time: 40 minutes

Prep time: 10 minutes

Cook time: 30 minutes

Yield: 6 servings

Ingredients

- 2 tbsp. extra virgin olive oil, divided
- 6 skinless chicken breast halves, cut in half crosswise
- ½ cup Kalamata olives, pitted
- 1 tbsp. freshly squeezed lemon juice
- 1 1/2 pounds mustard greens , stalks removed and coarsely chopped
- 1 cup dry white wine
- 4 garlic cloves, smashed
- 1 medium red onion, halved and thinly sliced
- Sea salt
- Ground pepper
- Lemon wedges, for serving

Directions

- Heat 1 tablespoon of extra virgin olive oil in a Dutch oven or large heavy pot over medium high heat.
- Rub the chicken with sea salt and pepper and add half of it to the pot; cook, for about 8 minutes or until browned on all sides.

44

- Transfer the cooked chicken to a plate and repeat with the remaining chicken and oil.
- Add garlic and onion to the pot and lower heat to medium; cook, stirring, for about 6 minutes or until tender.
- Add chicken (with accumulated juices) and wine and bring to a boil.
- Reduce heat and cook, covered, for about 5 minutes.
- Add the greens on top of the chicken and sprinkle with sea salt and pepper.
- Cook, covered, for about 5 minutes more or until the greens are wilted and chicken is opaque.
- Remove the pot from heat and stir in olives and lemon juice.
- Serve drizzled with accumulated pan juices and garnished with lemon wedges.

Delicious Mediterranean Chicken

Total time: 55 minutes

Prep time: 25 minutes

Cook time: 30 minutes

Yield: 6 servings

Ingredients

- 2 tsp. extra virgin olive oil
- ½ cup white wine, divided
- 6 chicken breasts, skinned and deboned
- 3 cloves garlic, pressed
- ½ cup onion, chopped
- 3 cups tomatoes, chopped
- ½ cup Kalamata olives
- ¼ cup fresh parsley, chopped
- 2 tsp. fresh thyme, chopped
- Sea salt to taste

Directions

- Heat the oil and 3 tablespoons of white wine in a skillet over medium heat.
- Add the chicken and cook for about 6 minutes on each side until golden.
- Remove the chicken and put it on a plate.
- Add garlic and onions in the skillet and sauté for about 3 minutes and add the tomatoes.
- Let them cook for five minutes then lower the heat and add the remaining white wine and simmer for 10 minutes.

- Add the thyme and simmer for a further 5 minutes.
- Return the chicken to the skillet and cook on low heat until the chicken is well done.
- Add olives and parsley and cook for 1 more minute.
- Add the salt and pepper and serve.

MEDITERRANEAN SEAFOOD RECIPES

Roasted Fish

Total time: 40 minutes

Prep time: 10 minutes

Cook time: 30 minutes

Yields: 4 servings

Ingredients

- 1 tbsp. olive oil
- 1 (14-oz) can drained artichoke hearts
- 4 cloves garlic, crushed
- 1 green bell pepper, cut into small strips
- ½ cup halved pitted olives
- 1 pint cherry tomatoes
- 1 tbsp. fennel seed
- 1 ½ lb. cod, quartered
- 4 ½ tsp. grated orange peel
- 2 tbsp. drained capers
- ⅓ to ½ cup fresh orange juice
- A pinch ground pepper
- A pinch salt

Directions

- Preheat your oven to 450°F.
- Generously grease a 10×15-inch baking pan with 1 tablespoon olive oil.
- Arrange the artichoke hearts, garlic, bell pepper, olives, tomatoes and fennel seed in the prepared pan.

- Place the fish over the vegetables and top with orange peel, capers, orange juice, pepper and salt.

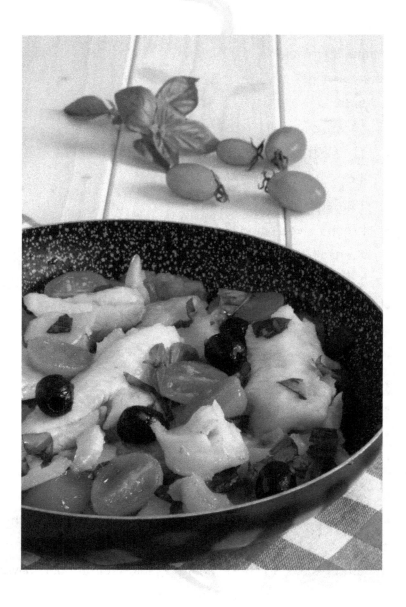

Baked Fish

Total time: 1 hour

Prep time: 10 minutes

Cook time: 50 minutes

Yields: 4 servings

Ingredients

- 2 tsp. extra virgin olive oil
- 1 large sliced onion
- 1 tbsp. orange zest
- ¼ cup orange juice
- ¼ cup lemon juice
- ¾ cup apple juice
- 1 minced clove garlic
- 1 (16 oz.) can whole tomatoes, drained and coarsely chopped, the juice reserved
- ½ cup reserved tomato juice
- 1 bay leaf
- ½ tsp. crushed dried basil
- ½ tsp. crushed dried thyme
- ½ tsp. crushed dried oregano
- 1 tsp. crushed fennel seeds
- A pinch of black pepper
- 1 lb. fish fillets (perch, flounder or sole)

51

Directions

- Add oil to a large nonstick skillet set over medium heat.
- Sauté the onion in the oil for about 5 minutes or until tender.
- Stir in all the remaining ingredients except the fish.
- Simmer uncovered for about 30 minutes.
- Arrange the fish in a baking dish and cover with the sauce.
- Bake the fish at 375°F, uncovered, for about 15 minutes or until it flakes easily when tested with a fork.

Spanish Cod

Total time: 35 minutes

Prep time: 20 minutes

Cook time: 15 minutes

Yield: 6 servings

Ingredients

- 1 tbsp. extra virgin olive oil
- 1 tbsp. butter
- ¼ cup onion, finely chopped
- 2 tbsp. garlic, chopped
- 1 cup tomato sauce
- 15 cherry tomatoes, halved
- ¼ cup deli marinated Italian vegetable salad, drained and chopped
- ½ cup green olives, chopped
- 1 dash cayenne pepper
- 1 dash black pepper
- 1 dash paprika
- 6 cod fillets

Directions

- Place a large skillet over medium heat and add the olive oil and butter.
- Add the onion and garlic and cook until garlic starts browning.
- Add the tomato sauce and tomatoes and let them simmer.
- Stir in the marinated vegetables, olives and spices.

- Cook the fillet in the sauce for 8 minutes over medium heat.
- Serve immediately.

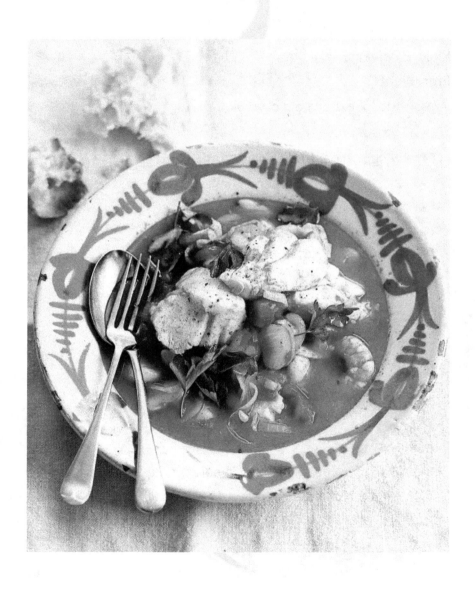

Greek Salmon Burgers

Total time: 30 minutes

Prep time: 15 minutes

Cook time: 15 minutes

Yield: 4 servings

Ingredients

- 1 pound skinless salmon fillets, diced
- 1 large egg white
- ½ cup panko
- 1 pinch sea salt
- ¼ tsp. freshly ground black pepper
- ½ cup cucumber slices
- ¼ cup crumbled feta cheese
- 4 (2.5-oz) toasted ciabatta rolls

Directions

- In a food processor, combine together salmon, egg white, and panko; pulse until salmon is finely chopped.
- Form the salmon mixture into four 4-inch patties and season with sea salt and pepper.
- Heat the grill to medium high heat and cook the patties, turning once, for about 7 minutes per side or until just cooked through.
- Serve with favorite toppings (such as sliced cucumbers and feta) and buns.

MEDITERRANEAN MEAT, BEEF AND PORK RECIPES

London Broil with Bourbon-Sautéed Mushrooms

Total time: 1 hour, 15 minutes

Prep time: 15 minutes

Cook time: 60 minutes

Yield: 3 servings

Ingredients

- ½ tsp. extra virgin olive oil
- ½ cup minced shallot
- ¾ lb. halved crimini mushrooms
- 6 tbsp. non-fat beef stock
- 3 tbsp. bourbon
- ½ tbsp. unsalted butter
- 1 tbsp. pure maple syrup
- Black pepper, to taste
- 1 lb. lean London broil
- ⅛ tsp. sea salt

Directions

- Preheat your oven to 400°F.
- Heat a nonstick skillet in oven for about 10 minutes.
- Remove and add extra virgin olive oil; swirl to coat the pan.
- Stir in shallots and mushrooms until well blended; return to oven and roast the mushrooms for about 15 minutes, stirring once with a wooden spatula.

- Stir in beef stock, bourbon, butter, maple syrup and pepper; toss and return the pan to oven; cook for 10 minutes more or until liquid is reduced by half.
- Remove pan from oven and set aside.
- Place another nonstick skillet in the oven and heat for about 10 minutes.
- In the meantime, sprinkle salt and ground pepper over the steak and place it in the hot pan.
- Roast in the oven for about 14 minutes, turning once.
- Remove the meat from oven and warm the mushrooms.
- Place steak on a cutting board and let rest for about 5 minutes.
- Thinly slice beef and serve top with sautéed mushrooms to serve.

Grilled Sage Lamb Kabob

Total time: 4 hours, 50 minutes

Marinating time: 4 hours

Prep time: 20 minutes

Cook time: 30 minutes

Yield: 2 servings

Ingredients

- 1 tbsp. fresh lemon juice
- 2 tbsp. fresh chives
- 2 tbsp. fresh flat leaf parsley
- 2 tbsp. fresh sage
- 1 tbsp. dark brown sugar
- 1 tbsp. extra virgin olive oil
- 2 tbsp. dry sherry
- 1 tbsp. pure maple syrup
- ¼ tsp. sea salt
- 8 ounces lean lamb shoulder
- 2 cups water
- 4 medium red potatoes
- White onion, cut into halves
- 6 shitake mushroom caps
- ½ red bell pepper

Directions

- In a blender, combine together lemon juice, chives, parsley, sage, brown sugar, extra virgin olive oil, sherry, maple syrup, and salt; puree until very smooth.

- Cut lamb into 8 cubes and add to a zipper bag along with the marinade; marinate in the refrigerator for at least 4 hours.
- Bring a pot with water to a rolling boil.
- Cut potatoes in halves and add to the pot along with half onion; steam for about 15 minutes. Remove from heat and let cool.
- Chop the remaining onion and pepper.
- On a skewer, alternate lamb cube, mushroom cap, pepper, onion and potato.
- Reserve the marinade.
- Grill the kabobs over hot grill, turning every 3 minutes and basting with the reserved marinade.

Lemony Pork With Lentils

Total time: 45 minutes

Prep time: 15 minutes

Cook time: 30 minutes

Chill time: 8 hours

Yield: 4 servings

Ingredients

- 2 tbsp. extra virgin olive oil, divided
- 4 (4 ounce) pork chops
- 2 tbsp. fresh lemon juice
- 1 tsp. lemon zest
- 1 clove garlic
- 2 tbsp. fresh rosemary
- 1 tbsp. parsley
- 1 tbsp. pure maple syrup
- 6 cups water, divided
- ½ cup green lentils
- 1 shallot
- 1 rib celery
- ½ cup dry sherry, divided
- 1 tsp. sea salt
- 1 tsp. unsalted butter
- ¼ tsp. red pepper flakes

Directions

- In a zipper bag, combine extra virgin olive oil, pork chops, lemon juice, lemon zest, garlic clove, rosemary, parsley, and maple syrup; refrigerate for at least 8 hours.
- Combine 3 cups of water and green lentils in a saucepan set over medium heat and cook for about 20 minutes or until lentils are just tender; drain and rinse.
- Preheat your oven to 350ºF.
- Heat a nonstick skillet over medium high heat and add the marinade; sear pork for about 2 minutes per side and transfer the skillet to the oven.
- In the meantime, heat 1 teaspoon of extra virgin olive oil to a second nonstick skillet set over medium high heat; add shallot, red pepper flakes and celery and lower heat to medium; cook for about 4 minutes or until tender. Stir in lentils until warmed through.
- Add ¼ teaspoon sea salt and ¼ cup sherry and cook for about 2 minutes or until liquid is reduced by half. Stir in butter until melted.
- Divide the lentil mixture among four plates and top each serving with one pork chop from first skillet.
- Remove and discard garlic from marinade in the first skillet and deglaze the pan with ¼ cup sherry; increase heat and stir in ¼ teaspoon sea salt; cook until the liquid is reduced by half.
- Evenly pour the sauce over each serving and serve.

Cumin Pork Chops

Total time: 30 minutes

Prep time: 10 minutes

Cook time: 20 minutes

Yield: 1 serving

Ingredients

- 4-ounce lean center-cut pork chop
- ⅛ tsp. sea salt
- ⅛ tsp. ground cumin
- Olive oil spray
- 2 tbsp. mashed avocado
- 2 tsp. fresh cilantro leaves

Directions

- Preheat your oven to 400°F.

VEGETARIAN AND LEGUMES MEDITERRANEAN RECIPES

Stewed Artichokes with Beans

Total time: 40 minutes

Prep time: 15 minutes

Cook time: 25 minutes

Yield: 4 servings

Ingredients

- 1 ½ pounds fava beans, shelled
- 3 tbsp. freshly squeezed lemon juice
- 4 cups water
- 24 baby artichokes
- 1 lemon half, to rub artichokes
- 2 tsp. extra virgin olive oil
- 4 sprigs fresh flat-leaf parsley
- 4 sprigs fresh thyme
- 1/4 tsp. crushed red-pepper flakes
- 1/4 tsp. freshly ground black pepper
- 1 tsp. sea salt
- 3 peeled and lightly crushed cloves garlic
- 1 lemon half, to rub artichokes

Directions

- Fill a large bowl with water and ice; set aside.
- Add water to a medium pot and bring to a rolling boil over high heat.
- Add fava beans and blanch for about 30 seconds.
- Remove the beans from hot water and add to a bowl with ice bath; let soak for about 5 minutes or until cold.

65

- Peel the skin from the fava beans and set aside.
- In a large bowl, combine lemon juice with 4 cups of water; set aside.
- Remove the tough outer leaves from the artichokes and cut off the tips.
- Trim each stem and peel; rub with the lemon half and place in the lemon-water mixture.
- Add extra virgin olive oil to a saucepan set over medium heat; heat until hot but not smoky.
- Add garlic, red pepper flakes, sea salt and black pepper; cook, stirring, for about 2 minutes or until the shallot is lightly browned.
- Stir in the artichokes, parsley, thyme, and 1 cup of lemon-water mixture; bring the mixture to a gentle simmer.
- Lower heat to medium low and continue simmering, covered, for about 14 minutes or until the artichokes are tender.
- Add the fava beans and continue cooking for 3 minutes more or until the beans are tender. Serve immediately.

Mediterranean Pasta with Olives, Tomatoes and Artichokes

Total time: 35 minutes

Prep time: 15 minutes

Cook time: 20 minutes

Yield: 4 servings

Ingredients

- 12 ounces whole-wheat spaghetti
- 2 tbsp. extra virgin olive oil, divided
- 2 garlic cloves, sliced
- ½ medium onion, thinly sliced lengthwise
- Coarse salt and ground pepper
- ½ cup dry white wine
- 1 artichoke heart, rinsed and cut lengthwise
- 1 pint grape or cherry tomatoes, halved lengthwise, divided
- ⅓ cup pitted Kalamata olives, cut lengthwise
- ½ cup fresh basil leaves, torn
- ¼ cup grated Parmesan cheese, plus more for serving

Directions

- Cook pasta in a large pot of boiling salted water following package instructions, until al dente; drain and reserve 1 cup of pasta water.
- Return the cooked pasta to the pot.

- In the meantime, heat 1 tablespoon of extra virgin olive oil; add garlic and onion, season with sea salt and black pepper and cook, stirring regularly, for about 4 minutes.
- Stir in wine and continue cooking for about 2 minutes more or until the liquid is evaporated.
- Stir in the artichoke and continue cooking for about 3 minutes more or until starting to brown.
- Stir in half of the tomatoes, and olives and cook for 2 minutes.
- Add pasta and stir in the remaining olive oil, tomatoes, basil and cheese; Add the reserved pasta water, as desired, to coat the pasta.
- Serve immediately with extra cheese.

Swiss Chard with Olives

Total time: 30 minutes

Prep time: 15 minutes

Cook time: 15 minutes

Yield: 4 servings

Ingredients

- 1 ¼ pounds trimmed and rinsed Swiss chard
- 1 tsp. extra virgin olive oil
- 2 garlic cloves, sliced
- 1 small yellow onion, sliced
- 1 jalapeno pepper, chopped
- ⅓ cup Kalamata olives (brine-cured), pitted and roughly chopped
- ½ cup water

Directions

- Separate stems from leaves of Swiss chard; cut the stems into small pieces and roughly chop the leaves; set aside.
- Heat extra virgin olive oil to a Dutch oven or a large skillet over medium heat.
- Add garlic, onion, and jalapeno; sauté for about 6 minutes or until onion is tender and translucent.
- Add olives, Swiss chard stems, and water and cook, covered, for about 3 minutes.
- Stir in the chard leaves and continue cooking, covered, for about 4 minutes or until the leaves and stems are tender.
- Serve immediately.

69

Grilled Veggies Tagine

Total time: 1 hour

Prep time: 10 minutes

Cook time: 50 minutes

Yield: 6 servings

Ingredients

- ¼ cup golden raisins
- 6 small red potatoes, cut in quarters
- ¼ cup pine nuts, toasted
- 2/3 cup couscous, uncooked
- 2 garlic cloves, pressed
- I medium red onion, wedged
- 1 tsp. fennel seeds, crushed
- ¼ tsp. cinnamon, ground
- 1 ¾ cups onions, chopped
- 1 tsp. extra virgin olive oil
- 1 tsp. cumin, ground
- ¼ cup green olives, pitted and chopped
- 1 ½ cups water
- ¼ tsp. freshly ground black pepper
- Cooking spray
- 2 red bell peppers, diced
- 1 green bell pepper, diced
- ½ tsp. kosher salt
- 2 tsp. balsamic vinegar
- ½ can tomatoes, chopped

Directions

- Prepare a gas or charcoal grill.
- Combine the bell peppers, red onion, and ¼ teaspoon sea salt, vinegar and ½ teaspoon olive oil in a zip lock plastic bag and toss well.
- Place a large nonstick saucepan on medium heat and add the remaining olive oil and add the garlic and chopped onion.
- Sauté these for about 3 minutes and add fennel, cumin and cinnamon.
- Let them cook for a further 1 minute then add the remaining salt, olives, raisins, potatoes, tomatoes, black pepper and water and bring the pan to a boil.
- Cover the saucepan, and simmer for 25 minutes or until the potatoes are tender
- Remove the onions and bell peppers from the plastic bag and grill on a rack coated with cooking spray for about 10 minutes.
- Boil the remaining water in a separate saucepan and slowly stir in the couscous.
- Remove from heat and cover the pan and let it stand for 5 minutes.
- Serve the tomato mixture over couscous and top with the grilled onions, bell peppers and pine nuts.
-
- Heat a large skillet over medium heat.

- In the meantime, season pork chop with sea salt and cumin.
- Spray the pan with extra virgin olive oil and add the seasoned pork chop.
- Place the pan in oven and cook for about 10 minutes, turn the pork chop over and spread the seared part with avocado.
- Return to oven and cook for about 10 minutes more or until pork is done.
- Serve pork garnished with cilantro over mashed potatoes.

MEDITERRANEAN
DESSERTS

CRÈME CARAMEL

Serves 12

- 5 cups whole milk
- 2 teaspoons vanilla extract
- 8 large egg yolks
- 4 large eggs
- 2 cups sugar, divided
- 1/4 cup water

Directions

- Preheat the oven to 350°F. Heat milk in a medium pot over medium-high heat to scalding (just below the boiling point). Remove from heat and add vanilla.
- Whisk eggs and 1 cup of sugar in a large bowl. Slowly whisk a ladle of milk into the eggs. Keep ladling milk, until all the milk is incorporated into the eggs. Let cool.
- Have twelve (3-inch) ramekins ready to fill. Bring remaining sugar and water to a boil in a small nonstick saucepan over medium-high heat. Reduce the heat to medium. Do not stir the sugar; gently swirl the pan instead. The water will evaporate and the sugar will darken and turn to caramel. Don't walk away from the pan because the sugar will burn quickly. When the sugar turns a dark golden caramel, remove the pan from the heat and divide the caramel evenly among the ramekins. Let the caramel harden.

- Distribute the custard evenly among the ramekins. Set ramekins in a large baking pan. Add hot water to pan until it reaches halfway up the side of the ramekins.
- Bake the custards for 25–30 minutes or until the custard is set. Carefully remove the ramekins from the water. Let the ramekins cool completely, and then refrigerate them for 8 hours or overnight.
- To serve the Crème Caramel, run a small knife around the edge of each ramekin and unmold it by inverting the ramekin over a dessert plate.

RICE PUDDING

Serves 12

- 2 1⁄2 cups long-grain rice, rinsed 9 cups whole milk, divided
- 1 large cinnamon stick, broken in two
- 3⁄4 teaspoon salt 1 tablespoon vanilla extract
- 3 (2-inch) strips lemon peel, pith removed
- 3 (2-inch) strips orange peel, pith removed
- 1 cup sugar
- 2 large egg yolks
- 1⁄2 cup raisins, soaked in 1 cup warm water 1 teaspoon ground cinnamon

Directions

- In a large pot over medium-high heat, combine the rice, 8 cups of milk, the cinnamon stick, salt, vanilla, lemon peel, orange peel, and sugar. Stir the mixture until the milk is scalding (just before boiling). Immediately reduce the temperature to medium-low. Cook the rice for 60–90 minutes or until the rice is cooked and the pudding has a creamy consistency. Stir occasionally to keep the rice from sticking to the bottom of the pot.
- Remove the cinnamon stick, lemon peel, and orange peel.
- Cook the remaining milk in a small pan over medium-high heat until scalded (just before boiling). In a small bowl, whisk the eggs thoroughly. Then slowly whisk a ladle of milk into the eggs. Keep ladling milk, one ladle at a time, until all the milk is incorporated into the eggs.

- Drain the raisins. Add the egg mixture and raisins to the rice pudding and stir to combine. Pour the pudding into a casserole dish and let it cool to room temperature. Cover and chill in the refrigerator for 8 hours or overnight.
- Serve the rice pudding at room temperature topped with a sprinkle of cinnamon.

BAKLAVA

Serves 16

- 2 1⁄4 cups sugar, divided 1 cup water
- 1⁄2 cup honey 1 tablespoon fresh lemon juice
- 2 cups walnuts
- 2 cups blanched almonds
- 1⁄2 teaspoon ground cloves
- 2 teaspoons ground cinnamon
- 3⁄4 cup white bread crumbs or ground melba toast 1 cup unsalted butter, melted
- 1 package phyllo, thawed, at room temperature

Directions

- Put 2 cups of sugar, water, and honey into a medium pot over medium-high heat. Bring the mixture to a boil, and then reduce the heat to medium-low and cook for 10 minutes. Add the lemon juice and cook for another 10 minutes. Allow the syrup to cool to room temperature.

- In a food processor, pulse the walnuts and almonds until they are finely crumbled. Transfer the nuts to a bowl and add the cloves, cinnamon, remaining sugar, and bread crumbs. Stir to combine and set it aside.

- Preheat the oven to 300°F. Brush the bottom and sides of a 9" × 13" baking pan with the melted butter.

- Cover the phyllo sheets with a damp towel so they don't dry out. Take a sheet, brush one side with butter, and lay it in the pan with a quarter of it hanging off the top edge.

Repeat for the bottom, left, and right edges of the pan. Place a fifth buttered sheet directly into the pan, so the entire bottom of the pan is covered.

- Sprinkle a third of the filling over the phyllo. Place four buttered sheets over the filling. Sprinkle another third of the filling over the sheets. Top the filling with another four buttered sheets. Sprinkle the remaining filling over the sheets. Top with four more buttered sheets. Fold in the hanging edges from the first four sheets and brush the entire surface with butter.

- With a sharp knife, score the top layers of phyllo, about 1/4-inch deep, into serving squares. The scoring will make the baklava easier to cut after it is baked. Bake the baklava for 90 minutes or until the phyllo is golden.

- Immediately after baking, ladle the syrup over the entire surface of the baklava. Use all the syrup. Let the baklava absorb the syrup as it comes to room temperature.

- Cut the baklava and serve at room temperature. Store uncovered at room temperature.

LEMON HALVA

Serves 10

- 4 cups water
- 2 cups sugar
- 8 (2-inch) strips lemon peel, pith removed
- 1/8 teaspoon ground cinnamon 1 cup plus 1 tablespoon unsalted butter, divided
- 2 cups coarse semolina flour
- 1/2 cup plus 2 tablespoons chopped blanched almonds, divided 1/2 cup plus 2 tablespoons pine nuts, divided 1/2 teaspoon vanilla 2 tablespoons grated lemon zest
- 2 tablespoons lemon juice

Directions

- Put the water, sugar, and lemon peels in a medium pot over medium-high heat. Bring the water to a boil, and then reduce the heat to medium-low and cook for 5 minutes. Add the cinnamon. Allow syrup to cool to room temperature. Remove the lemon peels and discard them. Set the syrup aside and reserve.
- Melt 1 cup of butter in a large pot over medium heat. Stir in the semolina with a wooden spoon and continue stirring for 5–6 minutes until the semolina is lightly toasted. Add 1/2 cup of almonds and 1/2 cup of pine nuts, and stir for 2 more minutes.
- To the pot, add the syrup and the vanilla, and reduce the heat to medium-low. Keep stirring for 2–3 minutes or until

the semolina absorbs the liquid and starts to come away from the sides of the pan. Take the pot off the heat. Add the lemon zest and juice. Place a tea towel over the pan, and then cover the pan with a lid to prevent a crust from forming on the halva. Cool for 10 minutes.

- Grease a bundt pan with the remaining butter. Spoon the halva into the pan and smooth out the top. Let the halva cool completely before unmolding it.
- Top the halva with the remaining almonds and pine nuts. Serve the halva at room temperature or cold.

MEDITERRANEAN BREAD

FETA AND HERB PULL-APARTS

Serves 12

Pizza Dough

- 1⁄4 cup all-purpose flour
- 3 cloves garlic, peeled and smashed
- 1⁄4 cup finely chopped scallions, ends trimmed
- 2 tablespoons chopped fresh parsley
- 1⁄2 teaspoon pepper, divided
- 1 1⁄4 teaspoons dried oregano, divided
- 1⁄2 teaspoon plus 1⁄8 teaspoon dried rosemary, divided
- 1⁄4 teaspoon plus 1⁄8 teaspoon red pepper flakes, divided
- 2⁄3 cup crumbled feta cheese
- 2⁄3 cup grated kasseri cheese or other sheep's milk cheese
- 1⁄4 teaspoon sesame seeds

Directions

- Let the dough rise in a warm place for 1 1⁄2–2 hours. Sprinkle flour on a clean work surface. Punch the dough down and tuck the outer edges inward; then place the dough on a floured work surface. Press your fingers down on the dough and spread it out. Divide the dough into 16–18 equal pieces and roll each piece into a ball. Cover the dough balls with a tea towel and let them rest.
- Process garlic, scallions, parsley, 1⁄4 teaspoon pepper, 1 teaspoon oregano, 1⁄2 teaspoon rosemary, and 1⁄4

teaspoon red pepper flakes in a food processor for 1 minute. Add the cheeses and pulse until smooth.

- Take one dough ball (keep the others covered) and press it into a 3-inch disc with the palm of your hand. Put 2 teaspoons of the cheese filling in the center and bundle the dough around the filling. Place the dough ball (seam-side down) in a greased, 14-inch round baking pan. Repeat with the remaining dough balls.
- In a small bowl, combine the remaining pepper, oregano, rosemary, red pepper flakes, and sesame seeds. Brush the tops of the dough with water and sprinkle with the herb mixture. Allow the dough to rise again in a warm place for 30 minutes. Preheat the oven to 400°F.
- Bake the dough on the middle rack for 30 minutes or until the top is golden. Let the bread cool for 10 minutes before removing it from the pan. Serve warm or at room temperature.

PONTIAKA PIROSKI

Serves 12

- 1½ teaspoons active dry yeast
- 1 teaspoon sugar
- 1½ cups tepid water ¾ cup plus
- 1 tablespoon extra-virgin olive oil plus extra for frying, divided
- 2½ teaspoons salt, divided
- 3½ cups all-purpose flour, divided 2 medium onions, peeled and finely chopped
- 4 scallions, ends trimmed and thinly sliced
- 4 large potatoes, cooked, skins peeled, and finely mashed
- 1 cup finely chopped fresh parsley
- ¼ cup finely chopped fresh mint
- ½ teaspoon pepper

Directions

- In a large bowl, combine the yeast, sugar, water, and ¼ cup oil. Set the mixture aside for 5 minutes. Stir in 1½ teaspoons salt. Spread ¼ cup flour on a work surface. Using a large wooden spoon or your hands, gradually stir 3¼ cups of flour into the yeast mixture. When the mixture comes together, empty the bowl onto the floured surface and knead until the dough is pliable and no longer sticks to your hands.
- Roll the dough into a ball and place it in a bowl. Rub the surface of the dough with 1 tablespoon of oil. Cover the

85

bowl with plastic wrap, and let the dough rise in a warm place until it doubles in size (1½–2 hours).

- Heat the remaining oil in a skillet over medium heat. Add the onions and scallions. Cook for 12–15 minutes or until the onions are light brown. Cool completely. In a medium bowl, combine onions and scallions, potatoes, parsley, mint, remaining salt, and pepper. Reserve.
- Pinch off a walnut-size piece of dough. Roll it into a ball and flatten it into a 3-inch disc. Place a tablespoon of filling in the center, and fold the dough over to create a half-moon shape. Pinch the ends to seal the filling into the dough. Repeat with the remaining dough and filling.
- Heat 3 inches of oil in a deep frying pan over medium-high heat until the oil temperature reaches 365°F. Fry the piroski for 2 minutes per side or until just golden. Transfer to a tray lined with paper towels. Serve them warm or at room temperature.

MEDITERRANEAN
RICE AND GRAINS

Mediterranean Orzo

Serves: 8

Ingredients

- 14 ounces orzo pasta
- 1 tablespoon Simple Truth™ Organic Italian Extra Virgin Olive Oil
- 1 jar (8.5 oz.) sun-dried tomatoes in oil, julienne cut
- 8 green onions, chopped
- 4 ounces feta cheese
- 1⁄4 cup provolone cheese, shredded
- 1 jar (16 oz.) Italian dressing

Directions

Step 1

Cook pasta in a large saucepan of boiling water with 1 tablespoon olive oil. Cook until done but still firm to bite. Drain and allow to cool.

Step 2

In a large bowl, combine pasta, sun-dried tomatoes, green onions, feta cheese and provolone. Pour dressing over top. Stir to combine.

MEDITERRANEAN
EGGS RECIPES

Mediterranean flavored egg scramble

Ingredients

- 6 eggs
- 1/4 cup light sour cream
- 1/4 teaspoon kosher salt
- A few cracks of freshly ground black pepper
- 1/4 teaspoon garlic powder
- 1/2 teaspoon dry basil
- 1/2 teaspoon dry oregano
- 3/4 cup crumbled feta cheese
- 2 tablespoon diced roasted red peppers
- 2 tablespoon minced green onions
- Crepes or warm flour tortillas

Instructions

- Preheat a skillet over medium heat.
- Whisk the eggs, sour cream, salt, pepper, basil, oregano, and garlic powder together. Gently add in the crumbled feta cheese. When the skillet is hot, add 1 tsp. butter and then add the eggs and allow them to begin to set up and then scrape the bottom of the pan to allow the liquid parts to cook. Stir in the roasted red peppers and green onions. Cook eggs until the desired doneness is reached. Serve immediately. If desired, sprinkle with a little extra feta cheese and wrap the scrambled eggs in a crepes or warm flour tortillas.

MEDITERRANEAN BREAKFAST BAKE

Mediterranean Breakfast Tarts

- 1 17.3 ounce package frozen Puff Pastry, (2 sheets)
- 1/2 cup Red Bell Pepper, finely diced
- 1/2 cup Green Pepper, finely diced
- 1/2 cup Red Onion, finely chopped
- 1 2.25 ounce can sliced Black Olives, drained and rough chopped
- 1/4 cup chopped fresh Parsley
- 1/2 teaspoon Greek Seasoning Blend, plus a few dashes for garnish
- 4 ounces cows milk Feta Cheese, crumbled
- 8 Cherry tomatoes, quartered
- 8 eggs
- 1 egg white, whisked, for egg wash on pastry

Directions

- Preheat oven to 400 degrees and line two baking sheets with parchment paper.
- Allow puff pastry to thaw for 30 minutes. Roll pastry dough out just slightly on a floured surface, cut each sheet into 4 squares, place four squares of puff pastry on each baking sheet.
- Crimp the corners of the pastry squares together folding each side up slightly creating a shallow basket.
- Toss peppers, onion, black olives, parsley, cheese, and Greek seasoning together in a bowl. Divide filling into 8, measures to be approximately a scant 1/4 cup, place filling

into each pastry basket spread to cover. Place in preheated 400 degree oven for 10 minutes.

- Remove from oven and brush edges of pastry with egg white, then crack an egg into each basket, being careful to keep egg from running out. Give each egg a dash of Greek seasoning blend. Add cherry tomato quarters if desired. Return to oven and bake for another 10-12 minutes.
- Remove from oven and serve immediately.

Mediterranean Diet Recipe: Vegetable Omelet

- 1 tablespoon olive oil
- 2 cups thinly sliced fresh fennel bulb
- 1 Roma tomato, diced
- 1/4 cup pitted green brine-cured olives, chopped
- 1/4 cup artichoke hearts, marinated in water, rinsed, drained, and chopped
- 6 eggs
- 1/4 teaspoon salt
- 1/2 teaspoon pepper
- 1/2 cup goat cheese, crumbled
- 2 tablespoons chopped fresh dill, basil, or parsley

Directions

- Preheat the oven to 325 degrees. In a large ovenproof skillet, heat the olive oil over medium-high heat.
- Add the fennel and sauté for 5 minutes, until soft.
- Add in the tomato, olives, and artichoke hearts and sauté for 3 minutes, until softened.
- Whisk the eggs in a large bowl and season with the salt and pepper.
- Pour the whisked eggs into the skillet over the vegetables and stir with a heat-proof spoon for 2 minutes.
- Sprinkle the omelet with the cheese and bake for 5 minutes or until the eggs are cooked through and set.
- Top with the dill, basil, or parsley.

- Remove the omelet from the skillet onto a cutting board. Carefully cut the omelet into four wedges, like a pizza, and serve.

Mediterranean Egg Casserole

Ingredients

- 1 tablespoon vegetable oil
- 1/4 cup chopped red onion
- 1/2 cup chopped red bell pepper
- 1 tablespoon finely chopped garlic (about 4 cloves)
- 2 cups packed fresh baby spinach, coarsely chopped
- 6 cups cubed (1-inch) French baguette
- 1 1/2 cups crumbled feta cheese (6 oz)
- 1/2 cup shredded Parmesan cheese
- 1 jar (6 oz) Progresso™ marinated artichoke hearts, drained well and coarsely chopped
- 1/3 cup pitted kalamata olives, halved
- 1/4 cup sun-dried tomatoes packed in oil, drained, chopped
- 10 eggs
- 2 cups milk
- 1/2 teaspoon red pepper flakes
- 1/2 teaspoon salt
- 1/2 teaspoon pepper

Directions

- Prevent your screen from going dark while you cook.
- Heat oven to 350°F. Spray 13x9-inch (3-quart) baking dish with cooking spray. In 8-inch nonstick pan, heat vegetable oil over medium heat. Cook onion, bell pepper and garlic in oil 3 to 5 minutes, stirring frequently, until slightly

softened. Add spinach, and cook about 1 minute or until starting to wilt.

- In baking dish, layer half of the baguette, 1 cup of the feta cheese, 1/4 cup of the Parmesan cheese, the bell pepper mixture, artichokes, olives and sun-dried tomato. Layer remaining baguette, and top with remaining 1/2 cup feta cheese. In large bowl, beat eggs and milk with whisk; beat in pepper flakes, salt and pepper. Pour over bread mixture, pressing down slightly. Sprinkle with remaining 1/4 cup Parmesan cheese.
- Bake 40 to 45 minutes or until golden brown and center is just set. Let stand 15 minutes before serving.

Low Carb Yeast Bread for Bread Machine

This is the best homemade low carb yeast bread recipe that I have found that gets great results every time. Can be baked in a bread machine or the oven.

Ingredients

- 1 package dry yeast Rapid Rise/Highly Active
- ½ teaspoon sugar see note
- 1 ⅛ cup warm water (120-130°F) 265 grams
- 3 Tablespoons olive oil 35 grams
- 1 cup vital wheat gluten flour 150 grams
- ¼ cup oat flour 35 grams
- ¾ cup soy flour see note
- ¼ cup flax meal 35 grams
- ¼ cup coarse unprocessed wheat bran 15 grams
- 1 Tablespoon sugar see note
- 1 ½ teaspoons baking powder
- 1 teaspoon salt

Instructions

NOTE: for best results, use weights as measure.

1. Proof the yeast by mixing it with the sugar and water at the bottom of the bread machine loaf pan. (If it's not bubbling, the yeast is no longer active so it should be tossed out)

2. Combine the oil, vital wheat gluten flour, oat flour, soy flour, flax meal, wheat bran, sweetener, baking powder, and salt in a medium bowl. Pour the dry mixture over the wet ingredients in the bread machine pan.

3. Set bread machine to the basic cycle (3-4 hours) and bake.
4. Cool on a rack then slice.

Notes

1. The original recipe called for sugar which should not contribute to the total carb count since it should be consumed by the yeast. So real sugar should be used if available.
2. Makes 16 slices. Nutritional data is per slice.
3. Almond flour should work as a substitute for soy flour as shown in the comments.
4. Proofing the yeast is optional. You can first add the wet ingredients into the pan and then add the combined dry ingredients with the yeast mixed in.
5. To make by hand, just combine the ingredients in a mixing bowl instead and knead for 8-10 minutes. Cover with a dishtowel and let the dough rise for an hour and a half. Then knead 4-6 times and place dough into an oiled pan. Cover again for about an hour then bake at 350°F for 30 to 40 minutes.

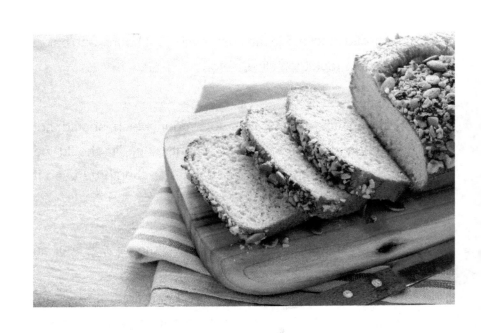